Healthy Smoothies Recipes

The ultimate healthy recipes to energize your days with delicious blends.

Maverick Slade

Table of contents

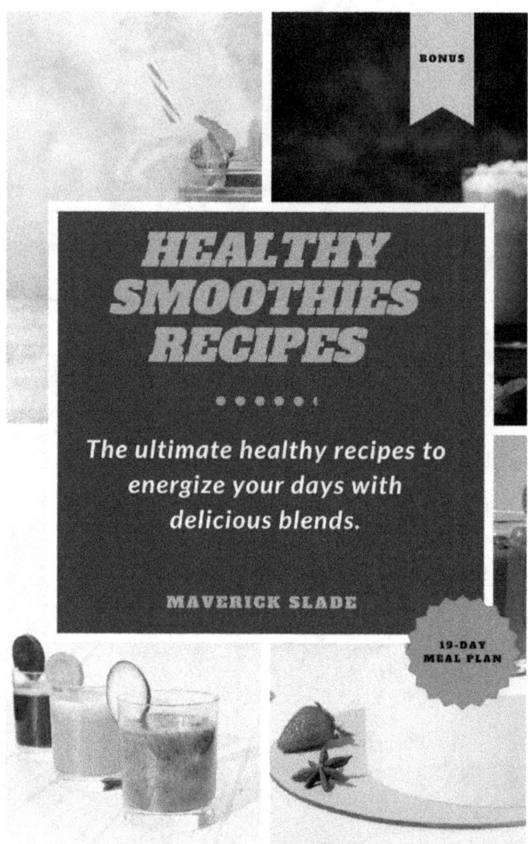
BONUS
HEALTHY
SMOOTHIES
RECIPES
The ultimate healthy recipes to
energize your days with
delicious blends.
MAVERICK SLADE
19-DAY
MEAL PLAN

Preface

Welcome to "Healthy Smoothie Recipes: Energize Your Day with Nutritious Blends"!

I am thrilled to share this collection of vibrant and nourishing smoothie recipes with you. In today's fast-paced world, finding time to prioritize our health can be challenging. That's why I've crafted this particular guidebook to make it easier for you to incorporate healthy habits into your daily routine.

Smoothies are not just drinks; they are power-packed meals in a glass, brimming with essential nutrients, vitamins, and minerals. Whether you're looking for a refreshing morning boost, a midday pick-me-up, or a calming evening treat, this book has you covered with up to 85 carefully curated recipes.

But this book is more than just recipes. It's a journey towards wellness, energy, and vitality. As you explore the pages ahead, you'll discover the countless benefits of incorporating smoothies into your diet. From increased energy levels to improved digestion and glowing skin, each sip brings you closer to a healthier and happier you.

I want to express my gratitude to all the health enthusiasts, nutritionists, and culinary experts whose knowledge and expertise have contributed to the creation of this guide. I also extend my heartfelt thanks to you, dear reader, for choosing this book to embark on your journey towards a healthier lifestyle.

Warmest regards.

Introduction to Healthy Smoothies

In a world where convenience often trumps nutrition, it's easy to overlook the importance of wholesome, nutrient-rich foods. However, with the rise of health-conscious living, more people are turning to simple yet powerful solutions to fuel their bodies and minds. One such solution? Healthy smoothies.

This guidebook is your gateway to a world of delicious and nutritious smoothie recipes designed to energize your day and nourish your body from the inside out. But before we delve into the recipes, let's take a moment to understand why smoothies have become a staple in the diets of health enthusiasts worldwide.

The Power of Smoothies

Smoothies are more than just blended fruits and vegetables; they are a potent combination of essential nutrients that can revitalize your entire being. By blending whole ingredients into a harmonious concoction, smoothies offer a convenient and delicious way to boost your intake of vitamins, minerals, fiber, and antioxidants.

Benefits Beyond the Blender

The benefits of incorporating smoothies into your diet extend far beyond the simple act of drinking them. From increased energy levels and improved digestion to glowing skin and enhanced immune function, the nutrients in each smoothie work synergistically to support your overall health and well-being.

A Recipe for Success

This guidebook is not just about providing you with recipes; it's about empowering you to take charge of your health. Each recipe is thoughtfully curated to offer a balance of flavors, nutrients, and textures. Whether you're a seasoned smoothie enthusiast or just starting your journey, you'll find recipes tailored to suit your taste buds and dietary needs.

How to Use This Guide

Navigating through this guide is simple yet effective. The book is divided into four sections: Morning Energizers, Afternoon Boosters, Evening Relaxation Blends, and All Time Smoothies. Each section features 20 unique smoothie recipes along with key information such as ingredients, preparation time, health benefits, and step-by-step instructions.

Whether you're looking to kickstart your day with a burst of energy, stay focused and alert in the afternoon, or unwind and relax in the evening, there's a smoothie recipe waiting for you.

Morning Energizers

1. Sunrise Citrus Bliss

- **Ingredients:** Oranges, bananas, Greek yogurt, honey, chia seeds.
- **Health Benefits:** Packed with vitamin C for immune support, potassium for electrolyte balance, and probiotics for gut health.
- **Preparation Method:**

1. Peel and chop 2 oranges and 1 ripe banana.
2. Blend the fruits with 1/2 cup Greek yogurt, 1 tbsp honey, and 1 tbsp chia seeds until smooth.
3. Pour into a glass and garnish with a slice of orange.

2. Green Goddess Revival

- **Ingredients:** Spinach, pineapple, avocado, coconut water, ginger.
- **Health Benefits:** Rich in antioxidants, fiber, and healthy fats, promoting detoxification and glowing skin.
- **Preparation Method:**

1. Combine 1 cup spinach, 1 cup pineapple chunks, 1/2 avocado, 1 cup coconut water, and a small piece of ginger in a blender.
2. Blend until creamy and smooth.
3. Pour into a glass and enjoy the vibrant green goodness.

3. Berry Blast Awakening

- **Ingredients:** Mixed berries (strawberries, blueberries, raspberries), almond milk, banana, oats.
- **Health Benefits:** Antioxidant-rich blend for brain health, energy, and satiety.

- Preparation Method:

1. Blend 1/2 cup mixed berries, 1/2 cup almond milk, 1 ripe banana, and 2 tbsp rolled oats until smooth.

2. Pour into a glass and top with a sprinkle of additional berries and oats.

4. Mango Tango Delight

-Ingredients: Fresh mango, coconut milk, turmeric, cinnamon, hemp seeds.

-Health Benefits: Anti-inflammatory properties, tropical flavor, and omega-3 fatty acids for heart health.

- Preparation Method:

1. Peel and chop 1 ripe mango.

2. Blend the mango with 1 cup coconut milk, a pinch of turmeric, a dash of cinnamon, and 1 tbsp hemp seeds until creamy.

3. Pour into a glass and savor the exotic flavors.

5. Peachy Keen Vitality Booster

- Ingredients: Peaches, Greek yogurt, almond butter, honey, flaxseeds.

- Health Benefits: High in antioxidants, protein, and essential fatty acids for sustained energy and muscle recovery.

- Preparation Method:

1. Slice 2 ripe peaches and blend with 1/2 cup Greek yogurt, 1 tbsp almond butter, 1 tbsp honey, and 1 tbsp ground flaxseeds until smooth.

2. Pour into a glass and enjoy the creamy peach goodness.

6. Tropical Paradise Sunrise

- Ingredients: Pineapple, mango, banana, coconut water, lime juice.

- Health Benefits: Hydrating, rich in vitamin C, and electrolytes for a refreshing start to your day.

- Preparation Method:

1. Blend 1 cup pineapple chunks, 1/2 cup mango chunks, 1 ripe banana, 1 cup coconut water, and the juice of half a lime until smooth.

2. Pour into a glass and garnish with a lime slice.

7. Vanilla Almond Dream

-Ingredients: Almond milk, vanilla protein powder, almond butter, dates, cinnamon.

- Health Benefits: Protein-packed, satisfying, and naturally sweetened for lasting energy.

- Preparation Method:

1. In a blender, combine 1 cup almond milk, 1 scoop vanilla protein powder, 1 tbsp almond butter, 2 pitted dates, and a sprinkle of cinnamon.

2. Blend until creamy and frothy.

3. Pour into a glass and sprinkle a bit of cinnamon on top.

8. Cherry Berry Bliss

- Ingredients: Cherries, mixed berries, spinach, coconut water, hemp hearts.

- Health Benefits: Antioxidant-rich, hydrating, and a good source of plant-based protein and omega-3s.

- Preparation Method:

1. Blend 1 cup cherries, 1/2 cup mixed berries, a handful of spinach, 1 cup coconut water, and 1 tbsp hemp hearts until smooth.

2. Pour into a glass and enjoy the burst of berry goodness.

9. Golden Turmeric Elixir

- Ingredients: Turmeric, banana, ginger, coconut milk, black pepper.

- **Health Benefits:** Anti-inflammatory, immune-boosting, and aids in digestion and joint health.
  - **Preparation Method:**
  1. Blend 1/2 tsp turmeric powder, 1 ripe banana, a small piece of fresh ginger, 1 cup coconut milk, and a pinch of black pepper until well combined.
  2. Pour into a glass and sprinkle a little extra turmeric on top for garnish.

10. Apple Pie Delight
  - **Ingredients:** Apples, oats, cinnamon, almond milk, honey.
  - **Health Benefits:** Fiber-rich, comforting flavors, and promotes satiety and blood sugar balance.
  - **Preparation Method:**
  1. Chop 1 apple and blend with 1/4 cup rolled oats, a sprinkle of cinnamon, 1 cup almond milk, and 1 tbsp honey until smooth.
  2. Pour into a glass and dust with a bit more cinnamon on top.

11. Blueberry Spinach Power
  - **Ingredients:** Blueberries, spinach, banana, almond milk, protein powder.
  - **Health Benefits:** Rich in antioxidants, iron, and protein for muscle recovery and energy.
  - **Preparation Method:**
  1. Blend 1/2 cup blueberries, a handful of spinach, 1 ripe banana, 1 cup almond milk, and 1 scoop of your favorite protein powder until smooth.
  2. Pour into a glass and enjoy the vibrant purple hue.

12. Pumpkin Spice Morning Blend
  - **Ingredients:** Pumpkin puree, banana, almond butter, pumpkin spice mix, almond milk.

- **Health Benefits:**High in vitamin A, fiber, and healthy fats, reminiscent of fall flavors.
   - **Preparation Method:**
   1.Combine 1/2 cup pumpkin puree, 1 ripe banana, 1 tbsp almond butter, a sprinkle of pumpkin spice mix, and 1 cup almond milk in a blender.
   2.Blend until creamy and top with a dash of extra pumpkin spice.

13. Cocoa Peanut Butter Boost

   - **Ingredients:** Cocoa powder, peanut butter, banana, Greek yogurt, almond milk.
   - **Health Benefits:**Packed with protein, potassium, and a hint of chocolatey goodness.
   - **Preparation Method:**
   1. Blend 1 tbsp cocoa powder, 2 tbsp peanut butter, 1 ripe banana, 1/2 cup Greek yogurt, and 1 cup almond milk until smooth.
   2.Pour into a glass and indulge in this satisfying treat.

14. Citrus Mango Zing

   - **Ingredients:**Mango, orange, lemon juice, Greek yogurt, honey.
   - **Health Benefits:**Vitamin C-rich, refreshing, and tangy flavors to awaken your senses.
   - **Preparation Method:**
   1. Blend 1 cup diced mango, the juice of 1 orange, 1 tbsp lemon juice, 1/2 cup Greek yogurt, and 1 tbsp honey until well combined.
   2. Pour into a glass and enjoy the tropical citrus burst.

15. Matcha Green Tea Elixir

- **Ingredients**: Matcha powder, banana, coconut water, honey, spinach.

- **Health Benefits:**Antioxidant-packed, natural energy boost, and promotes detoxification.

- **Preparation Method:**

1. Combine 1 tsp matcha powder, 1 ripe banana, 1 cup coconut water, 1 tbsp honey, and a handful of spinach in a blender.

2. Blend until smooth and pour into a glass for a vibrant green start to your day.

16. Pineapple Coconut Sunshine

- **Ingredients:** Pineapple, coconut milk, banana, turmeric, honey.

- **Health Benefits:** Tropical flavors, anti-inflammatory properties, and immune-boosting benefits.

- **Preparation Method:**

1. Blend 1 cup pineapple chunks, 1/2 cup coconut milk, 1 ripe banana, a pinch of turmeric, and 1 tbsp honey until creamy.

2. Pour into a glass and feel the sunshine in every sip.

17. Minty Fresh Green Refresher

-**Ingredients:** Cucumber, mint leaves, lime juice, green apple, coconut water.

-**Health Benefits:** Hydrating, detoxifying, and refreshing for a burst of energy.

- **Preparation Method:**

1. Blend 1/2 cucumber, a handful of mint leaves, the juice of 1 lime, 1 green apple, and 1 cup coconut water until smooth.

2. Pour into a glass and garnish with a mint sprig.

18. Raspberry Beetroot Radiance

- **Ingredients:**Raspberries, beetroot, Greek yogurt, honey, almond milk.

- **Health Benefits:** Rich in antioxidants, supports heart health, and adds a vibrant color to your day.

- **Preparation Method:**

1. Blend 1/2 cup raspberries, 1 small cooked beetroot, 1/2 cup Greek yogurt, 1 tbsp honey, and 1 cup almond milk until well combined.

2. Pour into a glass and enjoy the berry-beet goodness.

19. Carrot Cake Morning Bliss

- **Ingredients:**Carrots, banana, walnuts, cinnamon, almond milk.

- **Health Benefits:**Beta-carotene for eye health, fiber-rich, and reminiscent of indulgent carrot cake flavors.

- **Preparation Method:**

1. Blend 1/2 cup grated carrots, 1 ripe banana, a handful of walnuts, a sprinkle of cinnamon, and 1 cup almond milk until creamy.

2. Pour into a glass and sprinkle some chopped walnuts on top.

20. Chia Berry Protein Burst

- **Ingredients:** Mixed berries, chia seeds, protein powder, almond milk, honey.

- **Health Benefits:** Protein-packed, omega-3 fatty acids, and a burst of fruity goodness.

- **Preparation Method:**

1. Blend 1/2 cup mixed berries, 1 tbsp chia seeds, 1 scoop protein powder, 1 cup almond milk, and 1 tbsp honey until smooth.

2. Pour into a glass and sprinkle extra chia seeds on top for added texture.

About the Morning Energizers

Attention

Start your day with a burst of energy and a smile on your face. Imagine waking up to a morning ritual that fuels your body and mind with everything you need to tackle the day ahead.

Interest

Our Morning Energizer smoothies are packed with vitamins, minerals, and antioxidants to kickstart your metabolism and keep you feeling vibrant and alert. Picture yourself blending a colorful, nutrient-dense smoothie that tastes as good as it makes you feel.

Desire

These smoothies are not just a breakfast choice; they are a lifestyle. They help improve digestion, boost your immune system, and provide sustained energy without the crash of caffeine.

Start your day with a nutrient-rich smoothie and watch your energy levels soar.

Action

Don't let another morning slip by feeling tired and sluggish. Embrace the power of our Morning Energizers and transform your mornings into a time of vitality and joy. Try one today and feel the difference from the very first sip!

Afternoon Boosters

1. Mango Pineapple Turmeric Delight
- **Ingredients:** Mango, pineapple, turmeric, coconut water, ginger.
- **Health Benefits:** Anti-inflammatory, digestive aid, and tropical flavors to refresh your afternoon.
- **Preparation Method:**

1 Blend 1 cup diced mango, 1/2 cup pineapple chunks, a pinch of turmeric, 1 cup coconut water, and a small piece of ginger until smooth.

2 Pour into a glass and garnish with a slice of mango.

2. Banana Berry Protein Punch
- **Ingredients:** Banana, mixed berries, protein powder, almond milk, spinach.
- **Health Benefits:** Protein-rich, antioxidant-packed, and a boost of energy for the afternoon slump.
- **Preparation Method:**

1 Blend 1 ripe banana, 1/2 cup mixed berries, 1 scoop protein powder, 1 cup almond milk, and a handful of spinach until creamy.

2 Pour into a glass and top with a few fresh berries.

3. Peach Mango Mint Cooler
- **Ingredients:** Peach, mango, mint leaves, coconut water, lime juice.
- **Health Benefits:** Hydrating, refreshing, and a burst of fruity flavors to invigorate your senses.
- **Preparation Method:**

1 Blend 1 ripe peach, 1/2 cup diced mango, a few mint leaves, 1 cup coconut water, and the juice of half a lime until well blended.

2. Pour into a glass over ice and garnish with a mint sprig.

4. Blueberry Avocado Bliss

- **Ingredients:** Blueberries, avocado, almond milk, honey, vanilla extract.

-**Health Benefits:** Creamy texture, omega-3 fatty acids, and antioxidant-rich blueberries for brain health.

- **Preparation Method:**

1. Blend 1/2 cup blueberries, 1/2 avocado, 1 cup almond milk, 1 tbsp honey, and a splash of vanilla extract until smooth.

2. Pour into a glass and enjoy the creamy goodness.

5. Pineapple Ginger Green Tea Refresher

- **Ingredients:** Pineapple, ginger, green tea, honey, spinach.

- **Health Benefits:** Antioxidants from green tea, digestion aid from ginger, and a tropical twist with pineapple.

- **Preparation Method:**

1. Brew a cup of green tea and let it cool.

2. Blend 1/2 cup pineapple chunks, a small piece of ginger, the cooled green tea, 1 tbsp honey, and a handful of spinach until well blended.

3. Pour into a glass over ice and enjoy the refreshing blend.

6. Strawberry Banana Coconut Refuel

- **Ingredients:** Strawberries, banana, coconut milk, almond butter, chia seeds.

- **Health Benefits:** Rich in potassium, fiber, and healthy fats for sustained energy and satiety.

- Preparation Method:

1. Blend 1/2 cup strawberries, 1 ripe banana, 1/2 cup coconut milk, 1 tbsp almond butter, and 1 tsp chia seeds until smooth.

2. Pour into a glass and garnish with a sprinkle of chia seeds.

7. Citrus Carrot Ginger Zest

- Ingredients: Oranges, carrots, ginger, coconut water, honey.

- Health Benefits: Immune-boosting vitamin C, beta-carotene, and digestive aid from ginger.

- Preparation Method:

1. Juice 2 oranges and grate 1 carrot.

2. Blend the orange juice, grated carrot, a small piece of ginger, 1 cup coconut water, and 1 tbsp honey until well combined.

3. Pour into a glass and enjoy the zesty goodness.

8. Chocolate Banana Almond Indulgence

- Ingredients: Cocoa powder, banana, almond milk, almond butter, dates.

- Health Benefits: Rich chocolate flavor, potassium from bananas, and natural sweetness from dates.

- Preparation Method:

1. Blend 1 tbsp cocoa powder, 1 ripe banana, 1 cup almond milk, 1 tbsp almond butter, and 2 pitted dates until creamy.

2. Pour into a glass and sprinkle a bit of cocoa powder on top.

9. Green Powerhouse Detox

- Ingredients: Kale, cucumber, green apple, lemon juice, coconut water.

- Health Benefits: Detoxifying greens, hydrating cucumber, and vitamin C boost from lemon.

- Preparation Method:

1. Blend a handful of kale, 1/2 cucumber, 1 green apple, the juice of 1 lemon, and 1 cup coconut water until smooth.

2. Pour into a glass and enjoy the cleansing properties.

10. Tropical Mango Basil Smoothie

- Ingredients: Mango, basil leaves, coconut milk, lime juice, honey.

- Health Benefits: Refreshing tropical flavors, antioxidant-rich basil, and hydrating coconut milk.

- Preparation Method:

1. Blend 1 cup diced mango, a few basil leaves, 1/2 cup coconut milk, the juice of half a lime, and 1 tbsp honey until well blended.

2. Pour into a glass and garnish with a basil leaf.

11. Pineapple Kiwi Green Goddess

- Ingredients: Pineapple, kiwi, spinach, coconut water, mint leaves.

- Health Benefits: High in vitamin C, iron-rich spinach, and refreshing mint for a revitalizing boost.

- Preparation Method:

1. Blend 1 cup pineapple chunks, 1 peeled kiwi, a handful of spinach, 1 cup coconut water, and a few mint leaves until smooth.

2. Pour into a glass and garnish with a sprig of mint.

12. Peach Basil Lemonade Smoothie

- Ingredients: Peaches, basil leaves, lemon juice, Greek yogurt, honey.

- Health Benefits: Vitamin C from peaches and lemon, refreshing basil, and protein-rich Greek yogurt.

- **Preparation Method:**

1. Blend 2 ripe peaches, a few basil leaves, the juice of 1 lemon, 1/2 cup Greek yogurt, and 1 tbsp honey until creamy.

2. Pour into a glass and enjoy the citrus-basil fusion.

13. Berry Oatmeal Powerhouse

- **Ingredients:** Mixed berries, oats, almond milk, almond butter, honey.
- **Health Benefits:**Fiber-rich oats, antioxidants from berries, and healthy fats from almond butter.
- **Preparation Method:**

1. Blend 1/2 cup mixed berries, 1/4 cup rolled oats, 1 cup almond milk, 1 tbsp almond butter, and 1 tbsp honey until smooth.

2. Pour into a glass and sprinkle some oats on top.

14. Coconut Mango Matcha Madness

- **Ingredients:** Mango, coconut milk, matcha powder, honey, Greek yogurt.
- **Health Benefits:**Matcha for sustained energy, tropical mango, and probiotics from Greek yogurt.
- **Preparation Method:**

1. Blend 1 cup diced mango, 1/2 cup coconut milk, 1 tsp matcha powder, 1 tbsp honey, and 1/4 cup Greek yogurt until creamy.

2. Pour into a glass and enjoy the matcha-mango fusion.

15. Cherry Almond Chia Delight

- **Ingredients:** Cherries, almond milk, almond butter, chia seeds, vanilla extract.
- **Health Benefits:** Omega-3s from chia seeds, antioxidant-rich cherries, and nutty goodness from almonds.

- Preparation Method:

1. Blend 1/2 cup pitted cherries, 1 cup almond milk, 1 tbsp almond butter, 1 tbsp chia seeds, and a splash of vanilla extract until well combined.

2. Pour into a glass and garnish with a cherry on top.

16. Banana Peanut Butter Crunch

- **Ingredients:** Banana, peanut butter, oats, almond milk, honey.

- **Health Benefits:** Protein-rich from peanut butter, fiber-filled oats, and potassium from bananas.

- **Preparation Method:**

1. Blend 1 ripe banana, 2 tbsp peanut butter, 2 tbsp rolled oats, 1 cup almond milk, and 1 tbsp honey until smooth.

2. Pour into a glass and sprinkle some crushed peanuts on top for crunch.

17. Mint Chocolate Chip Delight

- **Ingredients:** Spinach, banana, cocoa powder, mint leaves, almond milk.

- **Health Benefits:** Antioxidants from cocoa, refreshing mint, and iron-rich spinach.

- **Preparation Method:**

1. Blend a handful of spinach, 1 ripe banana, 1 tbsp cocoa powder, a few mint leaves, and 1 cup almond milk until creamy.

2. Pour into a glass and add a few dark chocolate chips on top for a treat.

18. Pomegranate Blueberry Burst

- **Ingredients:** Pomegranate seeds, blueberries, Greek yogurt, honey, almond milk.

- **Health Benefits:** Antioxidant powerhouse, probiotics from Greek yogurt, and natural sweetness.

- **Preparation Method:**

1. Blend 1/2 cup pomegranate seeds, 1/2 cup blueberries, 1/2 cup Greek yogurt, 1 tbsp honey, and 1 cup almond milk until smooth.

2. Pour into a glass and garnish with a sprinkle of pomegranate seeds.

19. Apple Cinnamon Spice Smoothie

- **Ingredients:** Apple, cinnamon, oats, almond milk, maple syrup.

- **Health Benefits:** Fiber-rich apple, warming cinnamon, and a touch of sweetness from maple syrup.

- **Preparation Method:**

1. Blend 1 chopped apple, 1/4 tsp cinnamon, 2 tbsp rolled oats, 1 cup almond milk, and 1 tbsp maple syrup until well blended.

2. Pour into a glass and sprinkle a bit more cinnamon on top.

20. Carrot Ginger Orange Zinger

- **Ingredients:** Carrots, oranges, ginger, coconut water, honey.

- **Health Benefits:** Beta-carotene from carrots, vitamin C from oranges, and digestive aid from ginger.

- **Preparation Method:**

1. Blend 1/2 cup chopped carrots, the juice of 2 oranges, a small piece of ginger, 1 cup coconut water, and 1 tbsp honey until smooth.

2. Pour into a glass and enjoy the zesty zing.

About The Afternoon Boosters

Attention

Feeling that afternoon slump? It's time to recharge with an Afternoon Booster smoothie that revitalizes your energy and keeps you focused and productive.

Interest

Packed with superfoods and natural ingredients, our Afternoon Boosters provide a perfect pick-me-up. Imagine enjoying a smoothie that not only tastes amazing but also helps you power through the rest of your day with ease.

Action

Say goodbye to afternoon drowsiness and hello to sustained energy. Make our Afternoon Boosters a part of your daily routine and experience the productivity and focus you've been missing. Blend one up and conquer your day!

Evening Relaxation Blends

1. Banana Almond Butter Dream

- **Ingredients**: Banana, almond butter, almond milk, honey, cinnamon.

- **Health Benefits**: Potassium-rich banana, healthy fats from almond butter, and a touch of sweetness.

- **Preparation Method:**

1. Blend 1 ripe banana, 2 tbsp almond butter, 1 cup almond milk, 1 tbsp honey, and a sprinkle of cinnamon until creamy.

2. Pour into a glass and sprinkle a bit more cinnamon on top for flavor.

2. Chamomile Honey Lavender Calm

- **Ingredients**: Chamomile tea (cooled), honey, lavender extract, Greek yogurt, banana.

- **Health Benefits**: Relaxing chamomile, soothing lavender, and probiotics from Greek yogurt.

- **Preparation Method:**

1. Brew a cup of chamomile tea and let it cool.

2. Blend the cooled tea with 1 tbsp honey, a drop of lavender extract, 1/2 cup Greek yogurt, and 1 ripe banana until smooth.

3. Pour into a glass and enjoy the calming flavors.

3. Vanilla Coconut Chia Soother

- **Ingredients**: Coconut milk, vanilla extract, chia seeds, maple syrup, banana.

- **Health Benefits**: Omega-3s from chia seeds, creamy coconut milk, and natural sweetness from maple syrup.

- **Preparation Method:**

1. Mix 1 cup coconut milk, 1/2 tsp vanilla extract, 1 tbsp chia seeds, 1 tbsp maple syrup, and 1 ripe banana in a blender.

2. Blend until smooth and pour into a glass.

3. Let it sit for a few minutes to allow the chia seeds to thicken before enjoying.

4. Berry Lavender Serenity

- **Ingredients:** Mixed berries, lavender-infused honey, Greek yogurt, almond milk, lavender buds (for garnish).

- **Health Benefits:** Antioxidants from berries, calming lavender, and probiotics from Greek yogurt.

- **Preparation Method:**

1. Blend 1/2 cup mixed berries, 1 tbsp lavender-infused honey, 1/2 cup Greek yogurt, and 1 cup almond milk until creamy.

2. Pour into a glass and garnish with a sprinkle of lavender buds.

5. Soothing Pumpkin Spice Latte

- **Ingredients:** Pumpkin puree, espresso (cooled), almond milk, pumpkin spice mix, maple syrup.

- **Health Benefits:** Rich in antioxidants, warming spices, and a hint of caffeine for a cozy evening treat.

- **Preparation Method:**

1. Mix 1/4 cup pumpkin puree, 1/2 cup cooled espresso, 1 cup almond milk, 1/4 tsp pumpkin spice mix, and 1 tbsp maple syrup in a blender.

2. Blend until smooth and pour into a glass.

3. Optional: Sprinkle a bit of pumpkin spice on top for garnish.

6. Golden Turmeric Bedtime Elixir

- **Ingredients:** Turmeric powder, almond milk, honey, ginger, cinnamon.
- **Health Benefits:** Anti-inflammatory properties, calming spices, and aids in relaxation for bedtime.
- **Preparation Method:**

1. Warm 1 cup almond milk on the stove.

2. Stir in 1/2 tsp turmeric powder, 1 tbsp honey, a small piece of grated ginger, and a sprinkle of cinnamon.

3. Pour into a mug and sip slowly before bedtime.

7. Coconut Mango Sleep Smoothie

- **Ingredients:** Coconut water, mango, banana, coconut flakes, honey.
- **Health Benefits:** Hydrating coconut water, tropical mango, and natural sweetness for a soothing bedtime treat.
- **Preparation Method:**

1. Blend 1 cup coconut water, 1/2 cup diced mango, 1 ripe banana, 1 tbsp coconut flakes, and 1 tbsp honey until smooth.

2. Pour into a glass and garnish with a sprinkle of coconut flakes.

8. Blueberry Lavender Moonlight

- **Ingredients:** Blueberries, lavender extract, Greek yogurt, almond milk, maple syrup.
- **Health Benefits:** Antioxidants from blueberries, calming lavender, and probiotics from Greek yogurt.
- **Preparation Method:**

1. Blend 1/2 cup blueberries, a drop of lavender extract, 1/2 cup Greek yogurt, 1 cup almond milk, and 1 tbsp maple syrup until creamy.

2. Pour into a glass and enjoy the serene flavors.

9. Cherry Chamomile

- **Ingredients**: Cherries, chamomile tea (cooled), honey, Greek yogurt, almond milk.
- **Health Benefits**: Melatonin-rich cherries, calming chamomile, and probiotics from Greek yogurt.
- **Preparation Method**:

1. Brew a cup of chamomile tea and let it cool.

2. Blend 1/2 cup pitted cherries, the cooled chamomile tea, 1 tbsp honey, 1/2 cup Greek yogurt, and 1 cup almond milk until smooth.

3. Pour into a glass and enjoy the dreamy blend.

10. Spiced Carrot Cake Nightcap

- **Ingredients**: Carrots, cinnamon, nutmeg, almond milk, maple syrup.
- **Health Benefits**: Beta-carotene from carrots, warming spices, and natural sweetness from maple syrup.
- **Preparation Method**:

1. Blend 1/2 cup grated carrots, a sprinkle of cinnamon and nutmeg, 1 cup almond milk, and 1 tbsp maple syrup until well combined.

2. Pour into a glass and sprinkle a bit more cinnamon on top for garnish.

11. Ginger Turmeric Bedtime Soother

- **Ingredients**: Ginger, turmeric powder, almond milk, honey, black pepper.
- **Health Benefits**: Anti-inflammatory properties, aids in digestion, and promotes relaxation for bedtime.
- **Preparation Method**:

1. Warm 1 cup almond milk on the stove.

2. Add 1/2 tsp turmeric powder, a small piece of grated ginger, a pinch of black pepper, and 1 tbsp honey.

3. Stir well and pour into a mug to enjoy.

12. Banana Lavender Sleep Smoothie

- **Ingredients:** Banana, lavender extract, almond milk, Greek yogurt, maple syrup.
- **Health Benefits:** Relaxing lavender, potassium-rich banana, probiotics from Greek yogurt.
- **Preparation Method:**

1. Blend 1 ripe banana, a drop of lavender extract, 1/2 cup almond milk, 1/2 cup Greek yogurt, and 1 tbsp maple syrup until smooth.

2. Pour into a glass and enjoy the calming blend.

13. Cozy Vanilla Cinnamon

- **Ingredients:** Almond milk, vanilla extract, cinnamon, honey.
- **Health Benefits:** Warm flavors of vanilla and cinnamon, soothing for a good night's sleep.
- **Preparation Method:**

1. Heat 1 cup almond milk on the stove until warm.

2. Stir in 1/2 tsp vanilla extract, a sprinkle of cinnamon, and 1 tbsp honey.

3. Pour into a mug and savor the cozy flavors.

14. Pumpkin Spice Bedtime Bliss

- **Ingredients:** Pumpkin puree, cinnamon, nutmeg, almond milk, maple syrup.
- **Health Benefits:** Comforting pumpkin flavors, warming spices, and a touch of sweetness.

- Preparation Method:

1. Blend 1/4 cup pumpkin puree, a sprinkle of cinnamon and nutmeg, 1 cup almond milk, and 1 tbsp maple syrup until smooth.

2. Pour into a glass and sprinkle a bit more cinnamon on top for garnish.

15. Chocolate Cherry Sleepy Treat

- Ingredients: Cocoa powder, cherries, almond milk, Greek yogurt, honey.

- Health Benefits: Antioxidant-rich cocoa, melatonin from cherries, and protein from Greek yogurt.

- Preparation Method:

1. Blend 1 tbsp cocoa powder, 1/2 cup pitted cherries, 1 cup almond milk, 1/2 cup Greek yogurt, and 1 tbsp honey until creamy.

2. Pour into a glass and enjoy the chocolate-cherry goodness.

16. Berry Lavender Chamomile Smoothie

- Ingredients: Mixed berries, lavender-infused honey, chamomile tea (cooled), almond milk, Greek yogurt.

- Health Benefits: Antioxidants from berries, calming effects of lavender and chamomile, probiotics from Greek yogurt.

- Preparation Method:

1. Brew a cup of chamomile tea and let it cool.

2. Blend 1/2 cup mixed berries, 1 tbsp lavender-infused honey, the cooled chamomile tea, 1/2 cup almond milk, and 1/2 cup Greek yogurt until smooth.

3. Pour into a glass and enjoy the soothing blend.

17. Vanilla Chamomile Dream Smoothie

- Ingredients: Vanilla extract, chamomile tea (cooled), banana, almond milk, honey.

- **Health Benefits:**Calming effects of chamomile, potassium from banana, and natural sweetness from honey.
   - **Preparation Method:**
   1. Brew a cup of chamomile tea and let it cool.
   2. Blend the cooled chamomile tea with 1/2 tsp vanilla extract, 1 ripe banana, 1 cup almond milk, and 1 tbsp honey until creamy.
   3. Pour into a glass and enjoy the dreamy flavors.

18. Minty Melon Sleep Smoothie

   - **Ingredients**: Honeydew melon, mint leaves, almond milk, Greek yogurt, honey.
   - **Health Benefits:** Hydrating melon, refreshing mint, probiotics from Greek yogurt, and a touch of sweetness.
   - **Preparation Method:**
   1. Blend 1 cup diced honeydew melon, a few mint leaves, 1/2 cup almond milk, 1/2 cup Greek yogurt, and 1 tbsp honey until smooth.
   2. Pour into a glass and garnish with a mint sprig.

19. Lemon Lavender Blend

   - **Ingredients**: Lemon juice, lavender extract, almond milk, Greek yogurt, honey.
   - **Health Benefits:** Vitamin C from lemon, calming lavender, probiotics from Greek yogurt.
   - **Preparation Method:**
   1. Blend the juice of 1 lemon, a drop of lavender extract, 1 cup almond milk, 1/2 cup Greek yogurt, and 1 tbsp honey until creamy.
   2. Pour into a glass and enjoy the citrus-lavender fusion.

20. Cherry Vanilla Bedtime Smoothie

- **Ingredients**: Cherries, vanilla extract, almond milk, Greek yogurt, maple syrup.

- **Health Benefits**: Melatonin from cherries, comforting vanilla, probiotics from Greek yogurt, and a hint of sweetness.

- **Preparation Method:**

1. Blend 1/2 cup pitted cherries, 1/2 tsp vanilla extract, 1 cup almond milk, 1/2 cup Greek yogurt, and 1 tbsp maple syrup until smooth.

2. Pour into a glass and savor the cherry-vanilla goodness.

About The Evening Relaxation Blends

Attention

Indulge in a guilt-free treat that satisfies your sweet tooth and helps you unwind after a long day. This Evening Relaxation Blends are the perfect way to end your day on a high note.

Interest

These smoothies are crafted to offer relaxation and satisfaction without the excess calories. Imagine enjoying a creamy, delicious smoothie that feels like a treat but supports your health goals.

All-Time Healthy Smoothie Recipes

Delicious 30 all-time healthy smoothie recipes that can be enjoyed at any time of the day:

1. Tropical Paradise Bliss

   - **Ingredients**: Pineapple, mango, coconut milk, banana, spinach.

   - **Health Benefits**: Vitamin C-rich, hydrating, and packed with essential nutrients.

   - **Preparation Method:**

   1. Blend 1 cup diced pineapple, 1/2 cup diced mango, 1/2 cup coconut milk, 1 ripe banana, and a handful of spinach until smooth.

   2. Pour into a glass and imagine yourself in a tropical paradise.

2. Minty Watermelon Refresher

   - **Ingredients**: Watermelon, mint leaves, lime juice, cucumber, coconut water.

   - **Health Benefits**: Hydrating, refreshing, and perfect for hot days.

   - **Preparation Method:**

   1. Blend 1 cup cubed watermelon, a few mint leaves, the juice of 1 lime, 1/2 cucumber, and 1 cup coconut water until well combined.

   2. Pour into a glass over ice and garnish with a mint sprig.

3. Cocoa Banana Almond Crunch

   - **Ingredients**: Cocoa powder, banana, almond milk, almond butter, oats.

   - **Health Benefits**: Chocolatey goodness, potassium from bananas, and protein-packed.

- Preparation Method:

1. Blend 1 tbsp cocoa powder, 1 ripe banana, 1 cup almond milk, 1 tbsp almond butter, and 2 tbsp rolled oats until creamy.

2. Pour into a glass and top with a sprinkle of crushed almonds.

4. Green Goddess Detox

- Ingredients: Kale, green apple, celery, cucumber, lemon juice.

- Health Benefits: Detoxifying greens, vitamin C boost, and aids in digestion.

- Preparation Method:

1. Blend a handful of kale, 1 green apple, 1 stalk of celery, 1/2 cucumber, and the juice of 1 lemon until smooth.

2. Pour into a glass and enjoy the green goodness.

5. Peach Raspberry Sunrise

- **Key Ingredients:** Peaches, raspberries, Greek yogurt, honey, almond milk.

- Health Benefits: Antioxidants, protein from Greek yogurt, and natural sweetness.

- Preparation Method:

1. Blend 1 cup sliced peaches, 1/2 cup raspberries, 1/2 cup Greek yogurt, 1 tbsp honey, and 1 cup almond milk until well combined.

2. Pour into a glass and garnish with a peach slice.

6. Blueberry Lemon Burst

- Ingredients: Blueberries, lemon zest, Greek yogurt, almond milk, honey.

- Health Benefits: Antioxidant-rich, vitamin C boost, and probiotics from Greek yogurt.

- **Preparation Method:**

1. Blend 1/2 cup blueberries, zest of 1 lemon, 1/2 cup Greek yogurt, 1 cup almond milk, and 1 tbsp honey until smooth.

2. Pour into a glass and enjoy the burst of flavors.

7. Vanilla Mango Coconut Cream

- **Ingredients:** Mango, coconut cream, vanilla extract, banana, almond milk.
- **Health Benefits:** Creamy texture, tropical flavors, and a touch of sweetness.
- **Preparation Method:**

1. Blend 1 cup diced mango, 1/4 cup coconut cream, 1/2 tsp vanilla extract, 1 ripe banana, and 1 cup almond milk until creamy.

2. Pour into a glass and feel like you're indulging in a dessert.

8. Cherry Berry Antioxidant Blast

- **Ingredients:** Cherries, mixed berries, spinach, almond milk, honey.
- **Health Benefits:** Antioxidants, iron-rich spinach, and natural sweetness from honey.
- **Preparation Method:**

1. Blend 1/2 cup pitted cherries, 1/2 cup mixed berries, a handful of spinach, 1 cup almond milk, and 1 tbsp honey until well blended.

2. Pour into a glass and enjoy the colorful blast.

9. Pineapple Turmeric Ginger Zinger

- **Ingredients:** Pineapple, turmeric powder, ginger, coconut water, honey.
- **Health Benefits:** Anti-inflammatory, digestion aid, and tropical flavors.
- **Preparation Method:**

1. Blend 1 cup diced pineapple, a pinch of turmeric powder, a small piece of ginger, 1 cup coconut water, and 1 tbsp honey until smooth.

2. Pour into a glass and feel the zing.

10. Oatmeal Cookie Dough Delight
- **Ingredients:** Rolled oats, banana, almond butter, cinnamon, almond milk.
- **Health Benefits:** Fiber-rich oats, potassium from bananas, and a hint of sweetness.
- **Preparation Method:**

1. Blend 1/4 cup rolled oats, 1 ripe banana, 2 tbsp almond butter, a sprinkle of cinnamon, and 1 cup almond milk until smooth.

10. Oatmeal Cookie Dough Delight
- **Ingredients** Rolled oats, banana, almond butter, cinnamon, almond milk.
- **Health Benefits:** Fiber-rich oats, potassium from bananas, and a hint of sweetness.
- **Preparation Method:**

1. Blend 1/4 cup rolled oats, 1 ripe banana, 2 tbsp almond butter, a sprinkle of cinnamon, and 1 cup almond milk until smooth.

2. Pour into a glass and enjoy the comforting flavors.

11. Spicy Avocado Lime Smoothie
- **Ingredients:** Avocado, lime juice, cilantro, jalapeño, coconut water.
- **Health Benefits:** Healthy fats from avocado, vitamin C from lime, and metabolism-boosting jalapeño.
- **Preparation Method:**

1. Blend 1/2 avocado, juice of 1 lime, a handful of cilantro, a small piece of jalapeño (to taste), and 1 cup coconut water until smooth.

2. Pour into a glass and enjoy the spicy kick.

12. Strawberry Coconut Bliss

- **Ingredients**: Strawberries, coconut milk, chia seeds, honey, Greek yogurt.

- **Health Benefits**: Antioxidants from strawberries, healthy fats from coconut milk, and omega-3s from chia seeds.

- **Preparation Method**:

1. Blend 1 cup strawberries, 1/2 cup coconut milk, 1 tbsp chia seeds, 1 tbsp honey, and 1/2 cup Greek yogurt until smooth.

2. Pour into a glass and savor the creamy delight.

13. Pear Ginger Detox Smoothie

- **Ingredients:**Pear, ginger, spinach, cucumber, lemon juice.

- **Health Benefits**: Hydrating, detoxifying, and vitamin C-rich.

- **Preparation Method**:

1. Blend 1 pear, a small piece of ginger, a handful of spinach, 1/2 cucumber, and the juice of 1 lemon until smooth.

2. Pour into a glass and enjoy the refreshing detox.

14. Papaya Mint Mojito

- **Ingredients**: Papaya, mint leaves, lime juice, coconut water, honey.

- **Health Benefits**: Digestive enzymes from papaya, refreshing mint, and hydrating coconut water.

- **Preparation Method**:

1. Blend 1 cup diced papaya, a few mint leaves, juice of 1 lime, 1 cup coconut water, and 1 tbsp honey until smooth.

2. Pour into a glass and enjoy the tropical flavors.

15. Apple Cinnamon Protein Smoothie

- **Ingredients**: Apple, cinnamon, protein powder, almond milk, oats.

- **Health Benefits**: Fiber from apples, protein boost, and a touch of warming cinnamon.

- **Preparation Method:**

1. Blend 1 chopped apple, 1/2 tsp cinnamon, 1 scoop protein powder, 1 cup almond milk, and 1/4 cup oats until smooth.

2. Pour into a glass and relish the apple-cinnamon goodness.

16. Blackberry Basil Smoothie

- **Ingredients**: Blackberries, basil leaves, Greek yogurt, almond milk, honey.

- **Health Benefits**: Antioxidants from blackberries, refreshing basil, and probiotics from Greek yogurt.

- **Preparation Method:**

1. Blend 1/2 cup blackberries, a few basil leaves, 1/2 cup Greek yogurt, 1 cup almond milk, and 1 tbsp honey until smooth.

2. Pour into a glass and enjoy the unique flavor combination.

17. Cantaloupe Cucumber Cooler

- **Ingredients**: Cantaloupe, cucumber, mint leaves, coconut water, lime juice.

- **Health Benefits**: Hydrating, refreshing, and low in calories.

- **Preparation Method:**

1. Blend 1 cup diced cantaloupe, 1/2 cucumber, a few mint leaves, 1 cup coconut water, and juice of 1 lime until smooth.

2. Pour into a glass and savor the refreshing blend.

18. Carrot Orange Ginger Smoothie

   - **Ingredients:** Carrots, orange juice, ginger, Greek yogurt, honey.

   - **Health Benefits:** Beta-carotene from carrots, vitamin C from orange, and digestive benefits from ginger.

   - **Preparation Method:**

   1. Blend 1/2 cup chopped carrots, 1 cup orange juice, a small piece of ginger, 1/2 cup Greek yogurt, and 1 tbsp honey until smooth.

   2. Pour into a glass and enjoy the zesty flavors.

19. Raspberry Almond Delight

   - **Ingredients:** Raspberries, almond milk, almond butter, Greek yogurt, honey.

   - **Health Benefits:** Antioxidants from raspberries, healthy fats from almond butter, and protein from Greek yogurt.

   - **Preparation Method:**

   1. Blend 1/2 cup raspberries, 1 cup almond milk, 1 tbsp almond butter, 1/2 cup Greek yogurt, and 1 tbsp honey until smooth.

   2. Pour into a glass and enjoy the nutty berry goodness.

20. Beet Berry Beauty

   - **Ingredients:** Beets, mixed berries, Greek yogurt, almond milk, honey.

   - **Health Benefits:** Detoxifying beets, antioxidants from berries, and probiotics from Greek yogurt.

   - **Preparation Method:**

   1. Blend 1/2 cup cooked and diced beets, 1/2 cup mixed berries, 1/2 cup Greek yogurt, 1 cup almond milk, and 1 tbsp honey until smooth.

   2. Pour into a glass and relish the vibrant flavors.

21. Green Apple Kiwi Cooler

 - **Ingredients**: Green apple, kiwi, spinach, cucumber, coconut water.

 - **Health Benefits**: Vitamin C from kiwi, detoxifying greens, and hydrating cucumber.

 - **Preparation Method:**

 1. Blend 1 chopped green apple, 1 peeled kiwi, a handful of spinach, 1/2 cucumber, and 1 cup coconut water until smooth.

 2. Pour into a glass and enjoy the refreshing green goodness.

22. Pineapple Coconut Chia Delight

 - **Ingredients**: Pineapple, coconut milk, chia seeds, Greek yogurt, honey.

 - **Health Benefits**: Hydrating, omega-3s from chia seeds, and probiotics from Greek yogurt.

 - **Preparation Method:**

 1. Blend 1 cup diced pineapple, 1/2 cup coconut milk, 1 tbsp chia seeds, 1/2 cup Greek yogurt, and 1 tbsp honey until smooth.

 2. Pour into a glass and enjoy the tropical delight.

23. Peanut Butter Banana Oat Smoothie

 - **Ingredients**: Peanut butter, banana, rolled oats, almond milk, honey.

 - **Health Benefits**: Protein from peanut butter, fiber from oats, and potassium from banana.

 - **Preparation Method:**

 1. Blend 2 tbsp peanut butter, 1 ripe banana, 1/4 cup rolled oats, 1 cup almond milk, and 1 tbsp honey until smooth.

 2. Pour into a glass and enjoy the creamy nutty goodness.

24. Tangerine Dream

- **Ingredients:**Tangerines, banana, Greek yogurt, almond milk, honey.
- **Health Benefits:** Vitamin C from tangerines, protein from Greek yogurt, and natural sweetness.
- **Preparation Method:**

1. Blend 2 peeled tangerines, 1 ripe banana, 1/2 cup Greek yogurt, 1 cup almond milk, and 1 tbsp honey until smooth.

2. Pour into a glass and savor the citrusy flavors.

25. Mango Lassi Smoothie

- **Key Ingredients:** Mango, Greek yogurt, cardamom, honey, almond milk.
- **Health Benefits:** Tropical flavors, protein from Greek yogurt, and a hint of exotic cardamom.
- **Preparation Method:**

1. Blend 1 cup diced mango, 1/2 cup Greek yogurt, a pinch of ground cardamom, 1 tbsp honey, and 1 cup almond milk until smooth.

2. Pour into a glass and enjoy the exotic delight.

26. Cucumber Mint Lemonade

- **Ingredients:** Cucumber, mint leaves, lemon juice, coconut water, honey.
- **Health Benefits:** Hydrating, refreshing, and vitamin C boost.
- **Preparation Method:**

1. Blend 1/2 cucumber, a few mint leaves, juice of 1 lemon, 1 cup coconut water, and 1 tbsp honey until smooth.

2. Pour into a glass and enjoy the refreshing lemonade.

27. Kiwi Spinach Green Smoothie

- **Ingredients:** Kiwi, spinach, banana, almond milk, honey.

- **Health Benefits:** Vitamin C from kiwi, iron-rich spinach, and natural sweetness.

- **Preparation Method:**

1. Blend 2 peeled kiwis, a handful of spinach, 1 ripe banana, 1 cup almond milk, and 1 tbsp honey until smooth.

2. Pour into a glass and enjoy the green goodness.

28. Cranberry Orange Blast

- **Ingredients:** Cranberries, orange juice, banana, Greek yogurt, honey.
- **Health Benefits:** Antioxidants from cran

berries, vitamin C from orange, and probiotics from Greek yogurt.

- **Preparation Method:**

1. Blend 1/2 cup cranberries, 1 cup orange juice, 1 ripe banana, 1/2 cup Greek yogurt, and 1 tbsp honey until smooth.

2. Pour into a glass and savor the zesty flavors.

29. Sweet Potato Pie Smoothie

- **Ingredients:** Cooked sweet potato, cinnamon, nutmeg, almond milk, honey.
- **Health Benefits:** Beta-carotene from sweet potatoes, warming spices, and natural sweetness.
- **Preparation Method:**

1. Blend 1/2 cup cooked sweet potato, a sprinkle of cinnamon and nutmeg, 1 cup almond milk, and 1 tbsp honey until smooth.

2. Pour into a glass and enjoy the pie-like flavors.

30. Pomegranate Power Smoothie

- **Ingredients**: Pomegranate seeds, Greek yogurt, spinach, almond milk, honey.

- **Health Benefits**: Antioxidants from pomegranate, iron from spinach, and probiotics from Greek yogurt.

- **Preparation Method**:

1. Blend 1/2 cup pomegranate seeds, 1/2 cup Greek yogurt, a handful of spinach, 1 cup almond milk, and 1 tbsp honey until smooth.

2. Pour into a glass and enjoy the powerful blend.

Tips for Customizing Your Smoothies

Creating your own smoothie recipes can be a fun and rewarding process. Here are some tips and tricks to help you customize your smoothies to match your taste preferences and nutritional needs.

1. Choose Your Base

The base of your smoothie is the liquid component that helps blend all the ingredients together. Here are some options:

- **Water:**Calorie-free and hydrating.
- **Milk:** Adds creaminess and protein (choose dairy or plant-based options like almond, soy, or oat milk).
- **Coconut Water:** Light and hydrating with a subtle tropical flavor.
- **Juices:** Adds sweetness and a punch of flavor (e.g., orange, apple, or pineapple juice).

2. Add Fruits and Vegetables

Fruits and vegetables are the core of any smoothie, providing flavor, nutrients, and natural sweetness. Here are some combinations to try:

- **Berries:** Strawberries, blueberries, raspberries, and blackberries are rich in antioxidants.
- **Tropical Fruits:** Pineapple, mango, and papaya add a sweet, exotic flavor.
- **Citrus:** Oranges, lemons, and limes add a zesty kick.
- **Greens:** Spinach, kale, and cucumber provide vitamins and a green color without overwhelming the flavor.
- **Root Vegetables:** Carrots and beets can add a sweet, earthy taste.

3. Boost with Protein

Adding protein to your smoothie helps keep you full longer and aids in muscle repair and growth. Consider these options:

- **Greek Yogurt**: Creamy texture and high in protein.
- **Protein Powders**: Whey, soy, or plant-based powders can be easily added.
- **Nut Butters**: Almond, peanut, or cashew butter adds creaminess and protein.
- **Silken Tofu**: A great vegan option that blends smoothly.

4. Enhance with Superfoods

Superfoods can give your smoothie an extra nutritional punch. Here are some popular choices:

- **Chia Seeds**: High in omega-3 fatty acids and fiber.
- **Flaxseeds**: Rich in fiber and healthy fats.
- **Hemp Seeds**: Provide protein, omega-3s, and omega-6s.
- **Spirulina**: A blue-green algae that's packed with nutrients.
- **Matcha Powder:** Adds a boost of antioxidants and a subtle green tea flavor.
- **Cacao** Nibs: For a chocolatey flavor and added antioxidants.

5. Sweeten Naturally

If you prefer a sweeter smoothie, consider these natural sweeteners instead of refined sugar:
- **Honey**: Adds a natural sweetness and has antimicrobial properties.
- **Maple Syrup**: A vegan option with a rich flavor.
- **Dates**: Blend well and add a caramel-like sweetness.
- **Stevia**: A zero-calorie, plant-based sweetener.

6. Incorporate Healthy Fats

Healthy fats can improve satiety and enhance the absorption of fat-soluble vitamins. Try these options:

- **Avocado**: Adds creaminess and healthy monounsaturated fats.
- **Coconut Oil**: Adds a subtle coconut flavor and medium-chain triglycerides (MCTs).
- **Nuts and Seeds**: Almonds, walnuts, chia seeds, and flaxseeds add crunch and nutrients.

7. Experiment with Spices and Extracts

Spices and extracts can add depth and complexity to your smoothie. Here are some to try:

- **Cinnamon**: Adds warmth and pairs well with fruits like apple and banana.
- **Ginger**: Adds a spicy kick and aids digestion.
- **Turmeric**: Provides anti-inflammatory benefits and a subtle earthy flavor.
- **Vanilla Extract**: Enhances sweetness and flavor without added sugar.
- **Mint**: Refreshing and pairs well with fruits like watermelon and berries.

8. Balance the Flavors

When creating your smoothie, aim for a balance of flavors—sweet, tart, and creamy. If your smoothie is too tart, add a bit of honey or banana. If it's too sweet, balance it with a splash of lemon juice or a handful of greens.

9. Texture Matters

Texture plays a crucial role in the enjoyment of your smoothie. Here are some tips to achieve the perfect consistency:

- **For a Thicker Smoothie**: Use frozen fruits, add a handful of ice, or include ingredients like oats or chia seeds.
- **For a Thinner Smoothie**: Add more liquid (water, milk, or juice) until you reach the desired consistency.

10. Plan Ahead

Making smoothies can be time-consuming, especially during busy mornings. Here are some tips for efficient smoothie prep:

- **Pre-Pack Ingredients**: Prepare and freeze smoothie packs with pre-measured fruits and vegetables. Just add your liquid base and blend.
- **Batch Prep**: Make a large batch of your favorite smoothie and store it in the fridge for up to 2 days, or freeze in portions for up to a month.
- **Use Fresh and Seasonal Ingredients**: Using fresh, seasonal produce not only enhances flavor but also maximizes nutritional benefits.

Summary

Customizing your smoothies allows you to tailor them to your taste preferences and nutritional needs. By experimenting with different bases, fruits, vegetables, proteins, superfoods, and spices, you can create endless combinations that are both delicious and nutritious. Enjoy the process of discovering your perfect blend.

Conclusion

As we come to the end of "Healthy Smoothie Recipes: Energize Your Day with Nutritious Blends," it's important to reflect on the journey we've taken together. This guidebook is more than just a collection of recipes; it's a celebration of health, wellness, and the simple joy of nourishing our bodies with nature's bounty.

Embrace the Journey to Health

Every smoothie you create is a step towards a healthier, more vibrant you. The beauty of smoothies lies in their versatility and the endless possibilities they offer. Whether you're looking to kickstart your day with a burst of energy, refuel after a workout, or simply enjoy a nutritious snack, there's a smoothie for every occasion.

Personalize Your Nutrition

We've explored a variety of recipes tailored to different times of the day, along with tips for customizing your smoothies to suit your personal tastes and nutritional needs. Remember, the best smoothie is the one that makes you feel good—inside and out. Don't be afraid to experiment and find the combinations that you love the most.

Nourish Your Body and Soul

Healthy eating is about more than just physical nourishment; it's about taking care of your whole self. As you blend your smoothies, take a moment to appreciate the vibrant colors, the fresh scents, and the nourishing ingredients. Let each sip be a reminder of your commitment to your well-being.

Stay Inspired

The world of smoothies is vast and ever-evolving. Stay inspired by exploring new ingredients, trying different flavor combinations, and continually learning about the nutritional benefits of various foods. Your smoothie journey is just beginning, and there's always something new to discover.

A Community of Wellness

By choosing to incorporate these healthy smoothie recipes into your daily routine, you're joining a community of wellness enthusiasts who value health, vitality, and the joy of living well. Share your creations with friends and family, inspire others with your journey, and enjoy the sense of community that comes from shared healthy habits.

Heartfelt Thanks

Thank you for allowing this guidebook to be a part of your wellness journey. Your commitment to health and your enthusiasm for exploring new ways to nourish your body are truly inspiring. May these recipes and tips bring you joy, health, and a renewed sense of energy each day.

Final Thoughts

In the hustle and bustle of daily life, it's easy to overlook the importance of taking care of ourselves. Let this guidebook serve as a gentle reminder to pause, blend, and savor the small moments of wellness. Here's to a healthier, happier you—one delicious smoothie at a time.

With heartfelt gratitude,

[Maverick Slade]

19-Day smoothies/meals plan

Days	Reviews	Remarks
1		
2		
3		
4		
5		
6		

7		
8		
9		
10		
11		
12		
13		
14		

15		
16		
17		
18		
19		

Please support us in dropping an honest review particularly on this book in other to reach out to more people looking for a book like this,and as well to also improve customer service experience.

9 798329 828856